Skin Picking

A Beginner's 7-Step Guide to Overcoming This and Other Body-Focused Repetitive Behaviors

copyright © 2024 Tyler Spellmann

All rights reserved No part of this book may be reproduced, or stored in a retrieval system, or transmitted in any form or by any means, electronic, mechanical, photocopying, recording, or otherwise, without express written permission of the publisher.

Disclaimer

By reading this disclaimer, you are accepting the terms of the disclaimer in full. If you disagree with this disclaimer, please do not read the guide.

All of the content within this guide is provided for informational and educational purposes only, and should not be accepted as independent medical or other professional advice. The author is not a doctor, physician, nurse, mental health provider, or registered nutritionist/dietician. Therefore, using and reading this guide does not establish any form of a physician-patient relationship.

Always consult with a physician or another qualified health provider with any issues or questions you might have regarding any sort of medical condition. Do not ever disregard any qualified professional medical advice or delay seeking that advice because of anything you have read in this guide. The information in this guide is not intended to be any sort of medical advice and should not be used in lieu of any medical advice by a licensed and qualified medical professional.

The information in this guide has been compiled from a variety of known sources. However, the author cannot attest to or guarantee the accuracy of each source and thus should not be held liable for any errors or omissions.

You acknowledge that the publisher of this guide will not be held liable for any loss or damage of any kind incurred as a result of this guide or the reliance on any information provided within this guide. You acknowledge and agree that you assume all risk and responsibility for any action you undertake in response to the information in this guide.

Using this guide does not guarantee any particular result (e.g., weight loss or a cure). By reading this guide, you acknowledge that there are no guarantees to any specific outcome or results you can expect.

All product names, diet plans, or names used in this guide are for identification purposes only and are the property of their respective owners. The use of these names does not imply endorsement. All other trademarks cited herein are the property of their respective owners.

Where applicable, this guide is not intended to be a substitute for the original work of this diet plan and is, at most, a supplement to the original work for this diet plan and never a direct substitute. This guide is a personal expression of the facts of that diet plan.

Where applicable, persons shown in the cover images are stock photography models and the publisher has obtained the rights to use the images through license agreements with third-party stock image companies.

Table of Contents

Disclaimer	3
Table of Contents	5
Introduction	7
Chapter 1: What is Skin Picking and BFRBs?	10
Symptoms that you Have a Skin Picking Disorder	10
Why Does Skin Picking Happen?	12
Chapter 2: Other Common BFRBs	17
Nail Biting (Onychophagia)	17
Hair Pulling (Trichotillomania)	18
Skin Picking (Dermatillomania)	19
Lip Biting and Cheek Chewing	20
Nose Picking (Rhinotillexomania)	21
Thumb Sucking	22
Scab Picking	23
Chapter 3: How to Treat Skin Picking Disorder and other BFRBs?	25
Therapy	25
Medication	27
Self-Help Strategies	28
Professional Help and Support Groups	29
Self-Care Practices	29
Managing Triggers and Maintaining Progress	30
Personalized Approach	31
Lifestyle Changes to Manage Skin Picking and Other BFRBs	31
Chapter 4: The Impact of BFRBs on Daily Life	33
Physical Health Implications	33
Emotional Well-being Implications of BFRBs	37
Social Interaction Implications of BFRBs	40

Productivity and Daily Functioning Implications of BFRBs 44

Chapter 5: The 7-Step Path to Recovery   **50**

Step 1: Awareness - Recognizing the Behavior   50

Step 2: Identification - Discovering Personal Triggers   53

Step 3: Education - Understanding the Disorder   56

Step 4: Replacement - Finding Alternative Behaviors   58

Step 5: Support - Seeking Help from Professionals and Support Groups   61

Step 6: Practice - Implementing New Habits Consistently   64

Step 7: Reflection - Monitoring Progress and Making Adjustments   66

Applying the 7 Steps to Other BFRBs   68

Chapter 6: Creating a Sustainable Routine for Lasting Change 71

Tips for Maintaining Progress and Preventing Relapse   71

Building a Supportive Environment and Lifestyle Changes   71

Emphasizing Self-care and Self-Compassion in the Recovery Journey   72

Conclusion   **73**

FAQ   **77**

What are Body-Focused Repetitive Behaviors (BFRBs) and how do they affect individuals?   77

What are the common triggers for BFRBs, and how can I identify mine?   77

What strategies can help in managing and reducing BFRBs?   77

How can mindfulness help in managing BFRBs?   78

What role does self-care play in managing BFRBs?   78

Are there any tools or apps that can assist in managing BFRBs? 78

What should I do if I experience setbacks in managing my BFRBs?   78

References and Helpful Links   **80**

More in this Series   **82**

Introduction

Did you know that skin picking, along with other Body-Focused Repetitive Behaviors (BFRBs) like hair pulling and nail biting, affects up to 5% of the population? These habits, often unnoticed, can escalate from minor annoyances to significant sources of stress and self-consciousness. They can affect both emotional well-being and physical health, remaining largely misunderstood by those who don't experience them.

In this guide, we will talk about the following;

- Understanding Skin Picking and BFRBs
- Identifying Symptoms of a Skin Picking Disorder
- Exploring the Causes of Skin Picking
- Discovering Other Common BFRBs
- Treating Skin Picking and Other BFRBs
- The Impact of BFRBs on Everyday Life
- Following the 7-Step Path to Recovery
- Building a Sustainable Routine for Long-term Change

What sets this guide apart is its holistic approach, addressing both the physical symptoms and emotional aspects of skin picking. It offers practical steps to reduce urges, promote healing, and nurture a positive mindset. This guide is like a toolkit, equipping you with the insights to identify triggers, manage stress, and develop healthier habits. Continue reading to discover the techniques and strategies that can help you overcome skin picking for good.

Chapter 1: What is Skin Picking and BFRBs?

Skin picking, also referred to as Dermatillomania or Excoriation Disorder, is classified as a Body-Focused Repetitive Behavior (BFRB). BFRBs encompass self-grooming actions that involve repeated pulling, picking, scratching, or biting directed at one's own body. These behaviors can vary in intensity from mild to severe and may involve focusing on the skin, nails, hair, or even teeth.

Body-Focused Repetitive Behaviors (BFRBs) are linked to obsessive-compulsive disorder (OCD) and are often performed as a way to alleviate stress or anxiety. Triggers can also include boredom, perfectionistic tendencies, or various emotional factors. While these behaviors may provide a temporary sense of satisfaction or relief, they can result in both physical harm and emotional distress in the long term.

Symptoms that you Have a Skin Picking Disorder

The symptoms of skin picking, or dermatillomania, can vary in severity but generally include the following:

1. **Visible Skin Damage**: This refers to noticeable sores, scars, or lesions on the skin that often result from repetitive picking. These marks can vary in size and

severity, frequently leading to further irritation or infection if not properly cared for.

2. **Frequent Picking**: This involves a persistent inability to resist the overwhelming urge to pick at the skin. Individuals may find themselves spending significant amounts of time engaged in this behavior, often without realizing how long they've been at it or how it affects their daily life.

3. **Attempts to Stop**: Many individuals make repeated but unsuccessful efforts to reduce or completely stop their skin-picking behavior. Despite wanting to change, they may struggle with breaking the habit due to its compulsive nature.

4. **Emotional Distress**: This includes experiencing feelings of shame, guilt, or embarrassment about the skin-picking behavior. These emotions can be powerful and may lead to additional mental health challenges, such as heightened anxiety or depression, impacting overall well-being.

5. **Avoidance of Social Situations**: Avoiding activities or situations where the skin damage might be visible to others, such as swimming or wearing certain types of clothing.

6. **Use of Tools**: Sometimes use tools like tweezers or pins to pick at the skin.

7. **Ritualistic Behavior**: Engaging in specific rituals or routines related to skin picking, such as picking in a particular order or pattern.

8. **Infections**: Recurrent skin infections due to open wounds and sores from picking.

These symptoms can significantly impact an individual's daily life, affecting their physical health, emotional well-being, and social interactions. Recognizing these symptoms is crucial for seeking appropriate help and treatment.

Why Does Skin Picking Happen?

The exact cause of skin picking is still not fully understood, but there are several factors that may contribute to its development and continuation. These include:

1. *__Psychological and Emotional Factors__*

- **Stress and Anxiety**

High levels of stress and anxiety are significant triggers for skin picking. Individuals may engage in this behavior as a coping mechanism to manage overwhelming emotions, finding temporary relief from the act of picking. This can provide a momentary distraction from their worries, but it often leads to a cycle of guilt and shame afterward, further perpetuating the behavior.

- **Obsessive-Compulsive Tendencies**

Skin picking often shares characteristics with Obsessive-Compulsive Disorder (OCD). Individuals may feel an uncontrollable urge to pick at their skin, leading to repetitive behaviors that are difficult to stop despite earnest efforts to cease. This compulsive nature can create a sense of frustration, as they may be aware of the harmful effects yet feel powerless to resist the urge.

- **Emotional Regulation**

For some, skin picking serves as a way to regulate emotions. The act of picking can provide a distraction from negative feelings or create a sense of control in a chaotic environment. It may become a ritualistic behavior, where individuals find solace in the repetitive motion, allowing them to temporarily escape from their emotional turmoil and regain a semblance of equilibrium amidst their struggles.

2. *__Environmental Influences__*

Situational Triggers

Certain environments or situations can significantly exacerbate skin picking behaviors. For instance, stressful settings, such as high-pressure work environments, academic pressures, or family conflicts, can heighten feelings of anxiety and discomfort.

This increased stress can lead individuals to resort to skin picking more frequently and with greater intensity, as a way to cope with their overwhelming emotions.

- **Learned Behaviors**

Skin picking often develops into a habitual response over time, closely tied to an individual's coping mechanisms. When a person repeatedly engages in this behavior, it can become reinforced through the temporary relief it provides from stress or anxiety.

As a result, skin picking may transform into a default response not only to emotional distress but also to specific environmental cues, such as being in a crowded place or during moments of boredom, making it increasingly difficult to break the cycle.

3. *__Habit Formation and Routine__*

- **Conditioned Response**

Over time, skin picking can evolve into a conditioned response, where the individual unconsciously engages in the behavior in reaction to specific triggers. These triggers can include emotions like anxiety, stress, or boredom, often leading to an automatic response that feels instinctive.

As the behavior becomes more entrenched, the person may find themselves picking their skin without even realizing it, which can create a cycle of shame and frustration.

- **Routine and Repetition**

The repetitive nature of skin picking can result in a deeply ingrained habit that is challenging to break. The brain starts to form associations between the physical act of picking and a sense of temporary relief or satisfaction, reinforcing the behavior. This cycle can become self-perpetuating, as the momentary ease experienced during skin picking can lead to repeated instances, making it increasingly difficult for the individual to recognize and address the underlying issues driving the behavior. These routines can significantly impact one's skin health, emotional well-being, and overall quality of life.

4. *<u>Genetic and Neurological Influences</u>*

- **Genetic Predisposition**

Research suggests that there may be a genetic component to skin picking, with individuals who have a family history of Body-Focused Repetitive Behaviors (BFRBs) being more susceptible to developing the behavior themselves.

Genetic studies indicate that certain hereditary traits could make some individuals more prone to impulsivity and anxiety, both of which are often linked to skin picking. This connection highlights the importance of understanding one's family medical history when assessing the risk of developing such behaviors.

- **Neurological Factors**

Research in neurobiology suggests that chemical imbalances in the brain, particularly involving neurotransmitters like serotonin and dopamine, could significantly contribute to skin picking behaviors. Serotonin is crucial for mood regulation, while dopamine is linked to the brain's reward system and impulse control.

Disruptions in the levels or functioning of these neurotransmitters can lead to increased anxiety and compulsive tendencies, potentially influencing the propensity for repetitive behaviors like skin picking. Understanding the neurological underpinnings of this behavior can help in developing targeted treatments and interventions.

Skin picking is a complex behavior arising from psychological, emotional, environmental, and biological factors. Understanding these causes is key to developing effective interventions and support for those affected. Addressing skin picking needs a holistic approach that considers mental health and environment, offering tools and support to manage and reduce the behavior.

Chapter 2: Other Common BFRBs

Apart from skin picking, there are other body-focused repetitive behaviors (BFRBs) that individuals may experience. These include:

Nail Biting (Onychophagia)

Nail biting is a prevalent Body-Focused Repetitive Behavior (BFRB) that involves the compulsive biting of one's nails, often leading to damaged nails and cuticles. This behavior is frequently triggered by stress, boredom, or anxiety and serves as a temporary distraction or stress relief.

Consequences: Chronic nail biting can result in painful and unsightly nails, increased risk of infections around the nail bed, and potential dental issues due to the constant pressure on teeth.

Coping Strategies:

- **Behavioral Interventions**: Regularly keep nails trimmed and well-manicured to reduce the temptation and opportunity to bite them. Consider applying a special bitter-tasting nail polish as a deterrent, which serves as a reminder whenever you unconsciously bring your nails to your mouth. This simple change in routine can gradually help in breaking the habit.

- **Stress Management**: Engage in a variety of stress-relieving activities such as regular exercise, deep breathing exercises, or meditation to address the underlying triggers that might lead to nail biting. These activities not only help reduce stress but also improve overall well-being, making it easier to manage impulses.

- **Alternative Activities**: Keep stress balls or fidget toys handy to provide an alternative outlet for nervous energy. These can keep your hands busy and effectively redirect the urge to bite nails into a healthier habit. Experimenting with different types of sensory toys can also be beneficial in finding what works best for you.

Hair Pulling (Trichotillomania)

Hair pulling involves the compulsive pulling out of hair from the scalp, eyebrows, or other body areas, often resulting in noticeable hair loss. It is typically used as a coping mechanism for stress or anxiety.

Consequences: This behavior can lead to bald patches, skin irritation, and significant emotional distress due to changes in appearance.

Coping Strategies:

- **Cognitive-Behavioral Therapy (CBT)**: Engage in sessions with a trained therapist to understand the psychological triggers behind hair-pulling urges. Together, you will work to identify these triggers and develop healthier coping mechanisms, which can help reduce or eliminate the behavior over time.

- **Habit Reversal Training**: This approach focuses on substituting hair pulling with a less harmful behavior. For instance, whenever the urge to pull hair arises, you can squeeze a stress ball or engage in an alternative activity that keeps your hands busy, helping to redirect the compulsion into a more positive action.

- **Mindfulness Techniques**: By practicing mindfulness, you can become more attuned to the moments when the urge to pull hair surfaces. Through mindfulness exercises such as meditation or focused breathing, you can learn to manage these urges more effectively, gaining greater control over the behavior and reducing its occurrence.

Skin Picking (Dermatillomania)

Skin picking involves picking at the skin, often leading to sores, scars, and infections. This behavior is triggered by stress, anxiety, or perceived skin imperfections.

Consequences: Chronic skin picking can cause severe skin damage, infections, and emotional distress due to visible scars.

Coping Strategies:

- **Skin Care Routines**: Establish and maintain a consistent skincare routine tailored to your skin type. This can help improve skin health and reduce the temptation to pick at perceived imperfections, as healthier skin often requires less attention.

- **Stress Management**: Incorporate various relaxation techniques, such as deep breathing exercises, meditation, or yoga, into your daily life. Effectively managing stress can significantly reduce the urge to pick, as stress often exacerbates the habit.

- **Barrier Methods**: Implement physical barriers like bandages or gloves to prevent skin picking. These barriers not only serve as a reminder to resist the urge but also physically block access to the skin, helping to break the cycle over time.

Lip Biting and Cheek Chewing

This behavior involves biting the inside of the lips or cheeks, causing sores and discomfort, often as a response to stress or anxiety.

Consequences: Repeated biting can lead to painful sores, infections, and changes in oral tissue.

Coping Strategies:

- **Mindful Awareness**: Develop a heightened awareness of the situations and times when nail biting occurs. Keeping a journal to track these instances can be beneficial in identifying patterns and triggers, ultimately helping to interrupt the habit.

- **Chewing Alternatives**: Consider using sugar-free gum or mints as alternatives to nail biting. These can satisfy the oral fixation without causing harm to your nails and fingers. Additionally, having these alternatives readily available can decrease the likelihood of resorting to nail biting.

- **Stress Reduction**: Engage in activities that are known to alleviate anxiety and stress, such as yoga, meditation, or deep breathing exercises. Regular practice of these activities can help reduce overall stress levels, which might be contributing to the nail-biting habit.

Nose Picking (Rhinotillexomania)

Nose picking involves compulsively picking the nose, which can lead to nasal damage and infections. It is often done out of habit or as a stress response.

Consequences: This behavior can cause nasal irritation, bleeding, and increase the risk of infections.

Coping Strategies:

- **Keep Hands Occupied**: Utilize stress-relief tools such as stress balls, fidget spinners, or even doodling to keep your hands busy. These activities can help reduce the urge to pick by providing an alternative focus and channeling nervous energy into something more productive.

- **Nasal Hygiene**: Regularly maintain nasal hygiene by using saline sprays or rinses to keep nasal passages moist. This practice helps alleviate dryness and irritation, which can often lead to picking. Additionally, consider using a humidifier in dry environments to ensure optimal moisture levels.

- **Awareness Techniques**: Engage in mindfulness exercises and practice self-awareness to recognize when the habit of picking is about to occur. By being conscious of the triggers and patterns, you can interrupt the behavior and replace it with healthier coping strategies. Meditation and breathing exercises can also be beneficial in fostering a more mindful approach.

Thumb Sucking

Common in children, thumb sucking involves sucking the thumb for comfort or stress relief, which can lead to dental issues if it persists into later childhood or adulthood.

Consequences: Prolonged thumb sucking can cause misalignment of teeth and affect oral development.

Coping Strategies:

- **Positive Reinforcement**: Implement a reward system to encourage children to stop sucking their thumbs by offering praise or small incentives, such as stickers or extra playtime, whenever they refrain from the habit. This positive feedback can motivate them to change their behavior over time.

- **Comfort Alternatives**: Introduce alternative comfort objects that children can use instead of thumb-sucking. Items such as a favorite soft toy, a cozy blanket, or even a stress ball can provide the emotional security and comfort they seek.

- **Habit Modification**: Apply bitter-tasting nail solutions to your child's nails to deter thumb-sucking. These harmless solutions create an unpleasant taste that discourages the behavior and helps children become more aware of when they are engaging in the habit.

Scab Picking

Similar to skin picking, scab picking involves picking at scabs, preventing healing and leading to scarring. It is often a response to stress or anxiety.

Consequences: This behavior can delay healing, cause infections, and result in permanent scars.

Coping Strategies:

- **Cover Scabs**: Use appropriate bandages or adhesive dressings to cover scabs, creating a physical barrier that helps reduce the temptation to pick and further irritate the healing area.

- **Moisturizing Routine**: Regularly apply a high-quality moisturizer to keep skin hydrated, which helps minimize itchiness and dryness. These conditions can often trigger the urge to pick, so maintaining a proper moisturizing routine is crucial for skin health and recovery.

- **Stress Management**: Engage in stress-relieving activities such as yoga, meditation, or deep-breathing exercises. These practices not only help manage stress but also address the underlying causes of compulsive picking behavior, promoting a healthier mindset.

Understanding these behaviors as coping mechanisms is critical in managing and reducing them. Recognizing the role of stress and anxiety can help in developing effective strategies to address these triggers and promote healthier habits.

Chapter 3: How to Treat Skin Picking Disorder and other BFRBs?

Body-Focused Repetitive Behaviors (BFRBs), including Skin Picking Disorder (Dermatillomania), are complex conditions that require a thoughtful and personalized approach to treatment. In this chapter, we will explore the various treatment options available for these conditions.

Therapy

1. **Cognitive Behavioral Therapy (CBT)**

Cognitive Behavioral Therapy (CBT) is a highly effective treatment approach for Body-Focused Repetitive Behaviors (BFRBs), such as skin picking. CBT works by helping individuals identify and change negative thought patterns that contribute to these behaviors.

Through techniques like cognitive restructuring, individuals learn to challenge and modify distorted thoughts, while behavioral interventions focus on developing healthier coping strategies. CBT addresses common triggers for BFRBs, such as stress and anxiety, by equipping individuals with tools to manage their emotional responses.

This therapeutic approach not only helps in gaining control over compulsive behaviors but also offers long-term solutions, greatly enhancing the quality of life for those affected.

2. **Habit Reversal Training (HRT)**

Habit Reversal Training (HRT) is an effective form of Cognitive Behavioral Therapy specifically designed to address Body-Focused Repetitive Behaviors (BFRBs) like skin picking. HRT works by first increasing the individual's awareness of their repetitive behavior, helping them recognize triggers and patterns.

The process involves awareness training, where individuals learn to identify the onset of their BFRB, followed by the development of a competing response—a new, incompatible habit that can replace the unwanted behavior.

Motivation enhancement is also a crucial step, encouraging individuals to stay committed to the change process. By focusing on these elements, HRT effectively reduces BFRBs and empowers individuals to better manage their behaviors, fostering healthier habits and improving overall quality of life.

3. **Mindfulness Techniques**

Mindfulness techniques are invaluable for individuals dealing with Body-Focused Repetitive Behaviors (BFRBs) by fostering a state of presence and heightened awareness. Practices like meditation and deep-breathing exercises are central to mindfulness, as they help reduce impulsivity and stress, common triggers for BFRBs.

By enhancing self-control and emotional regulation, mindfulness assists in breaking the habitual cycle associated with these behaviors. Engaging in regular mindfulness exercises promotes mental clarity and reduces anxiety, offering long-term benefits. Incorporating these practices into daily routines not only helps manage BFRBs but also contributes to a greater overall sense of well-being and emotional balance.

Medication

In some cases, medications may be prescribed to help manage the symptoms of BFRBs. These can include:

1. **Selective Serotonin Reuptake Inhibitors (SSRIs)**

Selective Serotonin Reuptake Inhibitors (SSRIs) are commonly prescribed medications for managing anxiety and depression, conditions that frequently co-occur with Body-Focused Repetitive Behaviors (BFRBs).

SSRIs function by increasing serotonin levels in the brain, which can help stabilize mood and reduce compulsive behaviors. This mechanism provides relief from the emotional distress often accompanying BFRBs and enhances overall mental health.

While SSRIs can be effective, it's crucial to use them under medical supervision to monitor side effects and efficacy. Combining SSRIs with therapeutic approaches like Cognitive Behavioral Therapy can offer a comprehensive treatment plan, addressing both the psychological and biological aspects of BFRBs.

2. **N-Acetylcysteine (NAC)**

N-Acetylcysteine (NAC) is an amino acid supplement that has gained attention for its potential in treating Body-Focused Repetitive Behaviors (BFRBs). NAC is thought to work by modulating glutamate levels in the brain, which may help in reducing the compulsive nature of BFRBs.

Some studies have shown promising results, indicating that NAC can decrease the severity of behaviors like skin picking and hair pulling. However, while the findings are encouraging, further research is needed to fully understand its efficacy and safety.

It's essential for individuals to consult healthcare professionals before beginning NAC supplementation, ensuring it's part of a comprehensive treatment strategy that may include therapy or other medications.

Medication should always be discussed with a healthcare provider to ensure it is appropriate and safe for the individual.

Self-Help Strategies

1. **Awareness and Tracking:** Keeping a journal to track episodes of BFRBs can increase awareness of patterns and triggers. This awareness is crucial for implementing effective changes.

2. **Alternative Behaviors:** Identify and practice alternative behaviors that can replace the BFRB. For example, using fidget toys or stress balls can help keep hands busy and redirect the urge.

3. **Environmental Modifications**: Make changes to the environment to reduce triggers. This could involve keeping areas clean to avoid the temptation of picking or organizing spaces to decrease stress.

Professional Help and Support Groups

1. **Therapists and Counselors:** Working with a mental health professional who specializes in BFRBs can provide structured support and guidance. They can tailor therapeutic approaches to fit individual needs.

2. **Support Groups:** Joining a support group offers a sense of community and understanding. Sharing experiences with others who face similar challenges can provide encouragement and practical advice.

Self-Care Practices

Self-care is a crucial aspect of managing Body-Focused Repetitive Behaviors (BFRBs). Establishing a balanced daily routine that includes regular exercise, healthy eating, and adequate rest can greatly enhance overall well-being and lower stress levels, a known trigger for BFRBs.

Incorporating mindfulness practices and relaxation techniques helps foster mental clarity and emotional stability. Engaging in hobbies and enjoyable activities provides an outlet for stress and enhances mood.

These self-care strategies not only support mental health but also build resilience and improve emotional regulation. By laying this foundation, self-care complements other therapeutic interventions, making it an essential part of a comprehensive management plan for BFRBs.

Managing Triggers and Maintaining Progress

1. **Identify Triggers:** Understanding what triggers the BFRB is critical. Common triggers include stress, boredom, and anxiety.

2. **Develop Stress Management Techniques:** Incorporate stress-relief activities such as yoga, meditation, or hobbies that you enjoy.

3. **Celebrate Progress:** Acknowledge and reward yourself for making progress, no matter how small. This positive reinforcement can motivate continued improvement.

Personalized Approach

Each individual's experience with BFRBs is unique, so treatment should be personalized. Combining different methods, such as therapy, medication, and self-help strategies, often yields the best results. Regularly reassess and adjust the treatment plan as needed to ensure it remains effective and aligned with personal goals.

By adopting a comprehensive approach to treating Skin Picking Disorder and other BFRBs, individuals can work towards managing their behaviors effectively and leading a healthier, more fulfilling life.

Lifestyle Changes to Manage Skin Picking and Other BFRBs

In addition to seeking professional treatment and practicing self-care, there are other lifestyle changes that can help manage BFRBs. These include:

- **Journaling:** Regularly writing down thoughts and emotions related to the Body-Focused Repetitive Behavior (BFRB) can provide valuable insight into personal triggers and patterns. This reflective practice helps individuals become more aware of the situations or feelings that lead to these behaviors, ultimately aiding in managing them more effectively.

- **Reminders or Visual Cues:** Placing reminders or visual cues in areas where picking frequently occurs can serve as a powerful tool to resist the urge. These cues can be anything from sticky notes with motivational messages to small objects that interrupt the habitual movement, helping to create a pause and redirect the behavior.

- **Reducing Access:** Limiting access to objects used for picking, such as tweezers, safety pins, or other tools, can significantly reduce temptation.

By keeping these items out of easy reach or replacing them with safer alternatives, individuals can decrease the likelihood of engaging in the behavior, promoting a healthier response to stress or anxiety.

Managing BFRBs requires patience, persistence, and a willingness to try different methods. With the right approach and support, it is possible to overcome these behaviors and improve overall well-being.

Chapter 4: The Impact of BFRBs on Daily Life

Now that we have discussed treatment and management of BFRBs, let's take a closer look at how these behaviors can impact daily life. BFRBs can affect an individual's physical, emotional, social, and occupational well-being.

Physical Health Implications

Body-Focused Repetitive Behaviors (BFRBs) can lead to a range of physical health challenges, each associated with specific behaviors. Understanding these repercussions provides insight into the broader impact on an individual's well-being.

1. ***Skin Picking (Dermatillomania)***

- **Skin Infections**

Chronic skin picking can break the protective skin barrier, making it more susceptible to frequent bacterial infections. These infections can range from minor irritations to serious conditions requiring medical treatment, and they can result in further skin damage, increasing the cycle of picking and infection.

- **Scarring and Tissue Damage**

Persistent skin picking can lead to deep skin lesions that heal poorly over time, resulting in permanent scarring and, in some cases, significant disfigurement. This can be particularly distressing for individuals, as it can dramatically affect their physical appearance and self-image, potentially leading to emotional and psychological challenges.

- **Impact on Healing**

The repetitive nature of skin picking can significantly interfere with the body's natural healing process. By continuously reopening wounds, it prolongs recovery time and increases the risk of complications such as infection or chronic sores, making it challenging for the skin to fully recover.

2. *__Hair Pulling (Trichotillomania)__*

- **Hair Loss and Scalp Damage**

Regular hair pulling can result in patchy hair loss, known as traction alopecia. This type of hair loss might become permanent if the damage to hair follicles is severe, as continuous tension weakens the follicle's ability to grow new hair. Over time, this condition can lead to visible bald patches that are often hard to conceal, potentially requiring medical treatments to address.

- **Infections and Irritation**

The repeated action of pulling hair can cause significant scalp irritation, as it creates small abrasions and weakens the skin's natural barrier. This irritation can increase susceptibility to infections, as bacteria and other harmful organisms have an easier time penetrating damaged skin. Such infections can lead to further discomfort and potential dermatological issues, sometimes necessitating medical intervention.

- **Psychological Impact**

The visible nature of hair loss can have a profound impact on a person's self-esteem and mental well-being. The appearance of bald patches can contribute to feelings of embarrassment and self-consciousness, leading to social anxiety and withdrawal from social interactions. This psychological impact can be as challenging to address as the physical symptoms, often requiring professional support to rebuild confidence and manage anxiety.

3. *__Nail Biting (Onychophagia) and Cheek Biting__*

- **Dental and Oral Health Issues**

Chronic nail biting can exert undue pressure on the teeth, potentially leading to misalignment or chipping of the enamel. Over time, this habit can also cause irritation and damage to the gums, increasing the risk of developing dental abnormalities such as malocclusion.

Additionally, the act of nail biting introduces bacteria from the nails into the mouth, heightening the likelihood of infections in the nail bed. Cheek biting, often accompanying nail biting, can create painful sores or ulcers inside the mouth. These can not only make eating and speaking uncomfortable but also become susceptible to bacterial infections if not properly managed.

- **Finger and Nail Bed Damage**

Engaging in continuous nail biting can result in sore, red fingertips due to the repetitive trauma inflicted on the skin around the nails. This can sometimes lead to bleeding, especially if the habit is severe or prolonged.

The repeated biting can affect the nail matrix, causing the nails to grow back in irregular or distorted shapes. Such changes may impact both the aesthetic appearance of the nails and their ability to perform everyday functions, like picking up small objects. Furthermore, damaged cuticles and open wounds around the nails can serve as entry points for pathogens, increasing the risk of infections and further complications.

The physical manifestations of BFRBs can profoundly affect an individual's self-esteem and confidence. Visible signs such as scars, bald patches, or damaged nails often lead to feelings of embarrassment and self-consciousness. Individuals may go to great lengths to hide these signs, impacting their social interactions and leading to a cycle of avoidance and isolation.

The physical health implications of BFRBs extend beyond immediate physical harm, contributing to broader psychological and social challenges. Addressing these behaviors comprehensively requires understanding both their physical and emotional dimensions.

Emotional Well-being Implications of BFRBs

The emotional impact of Body-Focused Repetitive Behaviors (BFRBs) is profound and multifaceted, affecting an individual's mental health and overall quality of life.

1. *Emotional Challenges*

- **Feelings of Shame and Guilt**

Individuals with Body-Focused Repetitive Behaviors (BFRBs) often experience intense feelings of shame about their behaviors. They might feel as though they lack control over their actions, which can be deeply distressing.

This shame is frequently coupled with guilt, particularly when they view their inability to stop as a personal failing. The overwhelming nature of these feelings can be pervasive, impacting their self-worth and leading to a continuous cycle of negative emotions that can be difficult to break without support or intervention.

- **Embarrassment**

The visible consequences of BFRBs, such as scars, bald patches, or damaged skin, can lead to significant embarrassment. Individuals may constantly worry about being judged or misunderstood by others, which can exacerbate feelings of isolation.

This fear often drives them to go to great lengths to conceal their behaviors, such as wearing long sleeves or hats, and to avoid social situations where they might be exposed. Consequently, the embarrassment associated with BFRBs can hinder their ability to engage fully in daily life and maintain healthy relationships.

2. ***Exacerbation of Anxiety and Depression***

- **Increased Anxiety**

Individuals dealing with Body-Focused Repetitive Behaviors (BFRBs) often face a heightened sense of anxiety. The persistent worry about being discovered or judged for their behaviors, such as hair pulling or skin picking, can significantly elevate anxiety levels.

This anxiety is not only a byproduct of the behaviors but often acts as a trigger, causing the individual to engage in these behaviors more frequently, thus perpetuating a vicious cycle that becomes increasingly difficult to break without intervention.

- **Depressive Symptoms**

The emotional and psychological toll of managing a BFRB can be profound. Constantly battling the urges to perform these habitual actions can lead to feelings of hopelessness and despair. The ongoing struggle to exert control over these behaviors, combined with the social isolation that frequently accompanies them due to fear of stigma or embarrassment, can contribute significantly to depression.

Individuals may find themselves experiencing a lack of motivation, an overwhelming sense of fatigue, or a diminished interest in activities they once found pleasurable, exacerbating their mental health challenges and creating additional barriers to seeking help.

3. *__Impact on Self-image and Mental Health__*

- **Negative Self-image**

The internalization of shame and guilt associated with Body-Focused Repetitive Behaviors (BFRBs) can severely damage an individual's self-image. Many people suffering from BFRBs perceive themselves as inherently flawed or broken, which can lead to a profound lack of confidence and persistent low self-esteem.

This negative self-perception often becomes a barrier to engaging in social and professional settings, exacerbating feelings of isolation. This isolation can further reinforce their negative self-view, creating a difficult cycle to break.

- **Potential for Mental Health Disorders**

The emotional and psychological challenges linked to BFRBs can develop into more serious mental health disorders. Anxiety and depression are common outcomes as individuals grapple with the stress of their compulsions and the resulting guilt or embarrassment.

In some cases, individuals may also experience obsessive-compulsive tendencies or body dysmorphic disorder, where they become excessively preoccupied with perceived flaws in their appearance. This preoccupation can lead to significant distress and impair daily functioning, further impacting their quality of life.

The emotional consequences of BFRBs are extensive, affecting every aspect of an individual's life. The persistent cycle of shame, guilt, and emotional distress can lead to severe mental health issues if left unaddressed.

Effective management of BFRBs requires a comprehensive approach that addresses both the physical and emotional dimensions, offering individuals the support and tools they need to improve their overall well-being and quality of life.

Social Interaction Implications of BFRBs

Body-Focused Repetitive Behaviors (BFRBs) significantly affect social interactions, creating barriers that can lead to a profound sense of isolation and affect personal relationships.

1. ***Impact of Visible Signs***

- **Physical Indicators**

The physical manifestations of Body-Focused Repetitive Behaviors (BFRBs), such as bald patches resulting from hair pulling (trichotillomania) or skin sores and scars from skin picking (dermatillomania), are often noticeable and can be difficult to conceal.

These visible signs not only attract unwanted attention but can also lead to intrusive questions and comments from others that individuals may find uncomfortable or distressing. This attention can exacerbate feelings of self-consciousness and shame, adding to the emotional burden of those struggling with BFRBs.

- **Self-consciousness**

The fear of being judged or misunderstood due to these physical indicators can lead to heightened self-consciousness and anxiety. Individuals may feel exposed or vulnerable in social settings, worried that others might notice their bald patches or skin damage.

This fear can severely impact their confidence, making them reluctant to participate in social activities or engage with others. As a result, individuals may choose to isolate themselves, avoiding situations where they might feel scrutinized, which can further affect their mental well-being and social life.

2. ***Social Withdrawal and Isolation***

- **Avoidance of Social Situations**

To protect themselves from potential judgment or embarrassment over their behaviors, individuals with Body-Focused Repetitive Behaviors (BFRBs) might withdraw from social activities. This avoidance can include skipping gatherings, not attending parties or public events, or even avoiding everyday interactions that others might take for granted, such as casual conversations or group activities. This protective mechanism, while understandable, can limit their exposure to positive social experiences.

- **Isolation**

This withdrawal can lead to a deep sense of isolation and disconnection from the social world. The lack of regular social interaction deprives individuals of the support, empathy, and connection that are vital for emotional well-being and personal growth.

This isolation can exacerbate feelings of loneliness, anxiety, and depression, contributing to a cycle of withdrawal that is difficult to break and can overall impact their quality of life and mental health.

3. ***Effects on Personal Relationships***

- **Strained Relationships**

The reluctance to engage socially can significantly strain existing relationships. Friends and family might not fully understand the underlying reasons behind the withdrawal, such as anxiety or fear of judgment, leading to feelings of frustration or resentment on both sides.

This can create a disconnect, making it difficult to maintain close bonds and potentially resulting in feelings of isolation and loneliness for the individual withdrawing.

- **Reduced Opportunities for Connection**

The fear of exposure to judgment or criticism, coupled with subsequent social withdrawal, can greatly reduce opportunities to form new and meaningful connections. This limitation not only affects personal friendships but also extends to professional relationships, which are crucial for networking and career advancement.

The absence of these connections can hinder access to diverse social support networks, impacting both emotional well-being and professional growth, and making it more challenging to navigate life's complexities.

4. ***Fear of Exposure and Avoidance***

- **Activity Avoidance**

The fear of exposing their Body-Focused Repetitive Behaviors (BFRBs) often leads individuals to avoid activities that might reveal their behaviors. This avoidance can include activities like swimming, where skin sores or bald patches might be visible, leading to embarrassment or unwanted questions from others.

It can also extend to professional settings, such as meetings or interviews, where personal appearance is scrutinized, and individuals might worry about being judged for their appearance.

- **Limitation of Experiences**

By avoiding these situations, individuals inadvertently limit their experiences and miss out on opportunities for growth, enjoyment, and connection with others. This restriction can lead to a narrower social world, as they might pass on social gatherings, sports, or recreational activities that could otherwise enrich their lives.

The constant self-consciousness and avoidance contribute to increasing feelings of being disconnected from society, potentially leading to isolation and impacting overall well-being.

The social implications of BFRBs are extensive, affecting an individual's ability to engage with others and maintain healthy relationships. Understanding these challenges is crucial for providing support and creating an empathetic environment where individuals feel safe to share their experiences and seek help. Encouraging open communication and fostering inclusive spaces can help mitigate these social barriers and improve the quality of life for those affected by BFRBs.

Productivity and Daily Functioning Implications of BFRBs

Body-focused Repetitive Behaviors (BFRBs) can significantly disrupt productivity and daily functioning, impacting various aspects of an individual's routine, work, and academic life.

1. ***Interference with Work and Study***

- **Time Consumption**

Engaging in Body-Focused Repetitive Behaviors (BFRBs) often consumes substantial amounts of time. For instance, an individual might spend hours each day on these behaviors, which can detract from important tasks and responsibilities.

This time-consuming activity leads to procrastination, causing delays in completing work or study-related activities. This can accumulate into significant setbacks in personal and professional goals.

- **Decreased Efficiency**

The distraction of managing or concealing BFRBs can significantly lead to decreased efficiency. Individuals dealing with BFRBs might find themselves unable to concentrate fully on their tasks, as their attention is frequently diverted by the urge to engage in these behaviors.

This lack of focus can result in lower-quality work, as well as missed deadlines, ultimately affecting their performance and productivity in both academic and professional settings.

2. *__Impact on Routine Management__*

- **Disruption of Daily Routines**

Regular engagement in Body-Focused Repetitive Behaviors (BFRBs) can significantly disrupt established routines, making it challenging to maintain a structured schedule. Individuals might find it difficult to stick to their daily plans due to unforeseen interruptions caused by these behaviors.

This disruption can lead to missed appointments, poor time management, and an overall feeling of chaos in day-to-day life, where even simple tasks become hurdles.

- **The Strain on Personal Life**

The compulsion to engage in repetitive behaviors often intrudes on valuable personal time, affecting an individual's ability to enjoy leisure activities or spend quality moments with family and friends.

This intrusion can create a work-life imbalance, where the person struggles to fulfill both personal and professional commitments. Over time, this can lead to feelings of guilt or isolation, as maintaining relationships and meeting responsibilities becomes increasingly difficult.

3. **_Psychological Toll and Fatigue_**

- **Emotional Exhaustion**

Constantly battling the urge to engage in Body-Focused Repetitive Behaviors (BFRBs) can lead to significant emotional exhaustion. This exhaustion stems from the persistent mental struggle to resist these urges, which often feels like a continuous uphill battle.

The stress and anxiety associated with these behaviors contribute to a deep sense of fatigue, not only reducing the energy available for other activities but also impacting one's overall mental well-being. Over time, this emotional depletion can affect relationships, work, and daily responsibilities, making it challenging to find enjoyment or fulfillment in everyday life.

- **Burnout**

The psychological toll of managing BFRBs can result in burnout. This state of burnout is characterized by feelings of being overwhelmed and emotionally drained by the relentless effort to control and manage the behaviors.

Individuals experiencing burnout may find themselves struggling with a lack of motivation and decreased performance across all areas of life, from professional responsibilities to personal interests. The constant struggle can also lead to a sense of frustration and helplessness, making it harder to pursue goals or engage in activities that were once enjoyable.

4. ***Effects on Career Progression and Academic Success***

- **Career Challenges**

In the workplace, the inability to focus and maintain productivity can significantly hinder career advancement. Individuals struggling with concentration issues may frequently miss out on promotions or key opportunities due to perceived unreliability, inefficiency, or a lack of commitment.

This can lead to stagnation in their career growth, affecting overall job satisfaction and long-term professional development.

- **Academic Implications**

For students, the impact of Body-Focused Repetitive Behaviors (BFRBs) can be particularly detrimental to academic success. These behaviors can lead to poor concentration, causing students to miss deadlines and reduce their active participation in academic activities, such as group projects and class discussions.

Consequently, this can result in lower grades and even academic probation, which may affect a student's confidence and future educational and career prospects. Addressing these challenges is essential to provide students with a supportive learning environment that fosters growth and achievement.

The challenges posed by BFRBs extend beyond immediate behavioral management, affecting the individual's ability to meet daily demands and responsibilities. Addressing these issues requires comprehensive support systems that provide coping strategies and accommodations in both educational and workplace environments.

By fostering understanding and offering tailored assistance, it is possible to mitigate the impact of BFRBs on productivity and help individuals achieve their personal and professional goals.

Despite these challenges, individuals with BFRBs often develop coping mechanisms to manage their behaviors. Strategies such as using fidget toys or wearing gloves can help keep hands occupied and reduce the frequency of behaviors.

Mindfulness and relaxation techniques like meditation and yoga can help mitigate stress and decrease the urge to engage in BFRBs. Therapeutic interventions, particularly Cognitive Behavioral Therapy (CBT) and Habit Reversal Training (HRT) are crucial in helping individuals understand their triggers and develop healthier coping strategies.

Chapter 5: The 7-Step Path to Recovery

If you're struggling with body-focused repetitive behaviors (BFRBs) like skin picking, nail-biting, or hair pulling, you're not alone. These behaviors often sneak into your routine without you realizing it, leading to both physical and emotional discomfort. The 7-step path to recovery is here to guide you toward overcoming these habits through awareness, understanding, and change.

Step 1: Awareness - Recognizing the Behavior

Body-Focused Repetitive Behaviors (BFRBs) are habitual actions that people may engage in without conscious realization, often as a response to stress, anxiety, or boredom. These behaviors can include actions like hair-pulling, skin-picking, or nail-biting. The first crucial step in addressing BFRBs is developing an acute awareness of when and why these behaviors occur.

1. **Keeping a Journal**

One of the most effective ways to become aware of your Body-Focused Repetitive Behaviors (BFRBs) is by maintaining a detailed journal. This doesn't just involve casual note-taking; it's about creating a comprehensive record that offers insights into your behavior patterns.

Regularly note down instances of the behavior, including the exact time, location, and any emotions or thoughts you were experiencing at that moment. Were you feeling stressed, bored, or anxious? Did something specific trigger the behavior?

This practice is instrumental in identifying patterns and pinpointing specific times of vulnerability. For instance, you might notice that your BFRBs occur more frequently during work or after a stressful meeting.

By consistently recording these details over a period of time, you create a valuable resource that can highlight triggers and recurring scenarios prompting the behavior. This not only aids in self-awareness but also provides crucial information that can be shared with a therapist or used to develop strategies for managing BFRBs.

2. **Recognizing Triggers**

Understanding the specific triggers of your Body-Focused Repetitive Behaviors (BFRBs) is essential for their effective management and long-term control. Triggers can vary widely from person to person, making it crucial to identify your unique set of circumstances.

Emotional states, such as stress, anxiety, or boredom, are common triggers.

Environmental factors can play a role, including being alone, in a particular setting, or even during specific times of the day. It's important to pay close attention to your emotional and physical state when a BFRB occurs.

This self-awareness allows you to anticipate and prepare for situations that may lead to these behaviors, enabling you to develop strategies to minimize their occurrence. By recognizing these patterns, you can take proactive steps to manage BFRBs more effectively and improve your overall well-being.

3. **Developing Mindfulness**

Mindfulness is a powerful tool in becoming aware of Body-Focused Repetitive Behaviors (BFRBs). By practicing mindfulness, you learn to focus your attention on the present moment, which can help you catch yourself before engaging in these habitual behaviors. This increased awareness allows you to identify the triggers and thoughts associated with BFRBs, providing an opportunity to intervene and choose a different response.

Techniques such as meditation, deep breathing, and body scans can significantly enhance your ability to stay present and aware. Through regular practice, these techniques can create a mental buffer against automatic responses, allowing you to pause and reflect before acting. By fostering a non-judgmental awareness of your actions and thoughts, mindfulness empowers you to make conscious decisions that promote healthier habits and well-being.

4. **Initiating Change**

Awareness is the key to initiating change. Once you have recognized your BFRBs and understood your triggers, you can begin to plan strategies to manage and reduce these behaviors. This might include developing alternative coping mechanisms, seeking support from professionals, or using behavioral interventions. The process of change begins with this foundational awareness, empowering you to take control and make positive adjustments in your life.

By dedicating time to observe and understand your BFRBs, you open the door to meaningful transformation and improved well-being.

Step 2: Identification - Discovering Personal Triggers

Identifying personal triggers for Body-Focused Repetitive Behaviors (BFRBs) is a critical step in managing and reducing these behaviors. Triggers can be diverse, and understanding them helps in creating effective strategies to cope with and mitigate BFRBs. Triggers are typically categorized into emotional, situational, and sensory, each playing a unique role in prompting these behaviors.

1. **Emotional Triggers**

Emotional triggers are internal states such as anxiety, stress, frustration, or even excitement that can lead to BFRBs. These feelings can create a sense of unease or restlessness, which individuals may subconsciously attempt to alleviate through repetitive behaviors.

To effectively identify emotional triggers, consider keeping a mood diary. Note the emotions you experience throughout the day and any corresponding BFRBs. Over time, patterns may emerge, revealing which emotions are most likely to trigger these behaviors.

2. **Situational Triggers**

Situational triggers are external circumstances or environments that can influence the occurrence of BFRBs. These might include specific locations, like being at home alone, or events such as stressful meetings or social gatherings.

To pinpoint situational triggers, reflect on where and when your BFRBs are most likely to occur. Consider the context and the presence of specific stressors in these environments. Understanding these patterns can help you anticipate and prepare for situations where you are more vulnerable.

3. **Sensory Triggers**

Sensory triggers involve physical stimuli that can provoke BFRBs. This might be the sensation of rough skin, an uneven nail, or even a strand of hair that feels out of place. These sensory cues can create an urge to engage in repetitive behaviors as a means of self-soothing or correction.

To identify sensory triggers, pay close attention to the physical sensations that immediately precede your behaviors. Mindfulness exercises and body scans can enhance your awareness of these sensory triggers, allowing you to recognize and address them more effectively.

4. **Developing Strategies for Management**

Once you have identified your personal triggers, you can begin to develop strategies to manage them. This might involve creating a plan to address emotional triggers through relaxation techniques or stress management.

For situational triggers, consider altering your environment or practicing coping strategies to minimize their impact. Sensory triggers might require adopting alternative responses, such as using fidget tools or practicing sensory grounding exercises.

Recognizing and understanding your personal triggers is pivotal in the journey to managing BFRBs. By acknowledging these triggers, you gain the insight needed to create personalized strategies that reduce the frequency and intensity of these behaviors. This self-awareness not only empowers you to break the cycle of BFRBs but also contributes to greater emotional and psychological resilience.

Taking the time to discover and understand your triggers opens the path to meaningful change and a healthier, more controlled approach to managing BFRBs.

Step 3: Education - Understanding the Disorder

Education is a powerful tool in managing Body-Focused Repetitive Behaviors (BFRBs). By gaining a deeper understanding of the disorder, you equip yourself with the knowledge to differentiate between misconceptions and reality. This awareness helps reframe BFRBs not as mere bad habits but as complex behaviors with psychological roots, paving the way for informed and effective coping strategies.

1. **Psychological Underpinnings of BFRBs**

BFRBs often have intricate psychological underpinnings. They may stem from underlying emotional issues such as anxiety, stress, or trauma. These behaviors can serve as coping mechanisms for dealing with complex emotions or as a means of self-soothing.

Understanding these psychological factors is crucial for recognizing that BFRBs are not simply the result of a lack of willpower but are connected to deeper psychological needs and responses.

2. **Benefits of Understanding BFRBs**

Educating yourself about BFRBs can significantly reduce feelings of shame and isolation. Recognizing that these behaviors are part of a recognized disorder can alleviate self-blame and help you view your actions with compassion rather than judgment.

This understanding fosters a sense of community and connection with others who experience similar challenges, breaking the isolation that often accompanies BFRBs.

3. **Informing Effective Coping Strategies**

Knowledge about BFRBs enhances your ability to choose effective coping strategies. By understanding the disorder, you can better assess which therapeutic approaches, whether behavioral therapy, mindfulness practices, or support groups, may work best for you.

Education empowers you to tailor interventions to your personal needs, increasing the likelihood of successful management and reduction of BFRBs.

4. **Reducing Shame and Isolation**

The journey of educating oneself about BFRBs also involves learning that you are not alone. Many people share similar experiences, and numerous resources and communities offer support and understanding. Engaging with educational materials, whether books, articles, or support networks, can provide reassurance and solidarity, reducing the stigma and shame often associated with BFRBs.

Embarking on an educational journey about BFRBs is a vital step towards healing and empowerment. By understanding the disorder, you can dismantle the myths surrounding these behaviors and approach them with empathy and informed action. This knowledge not only supports personal growth but also contributes to a broader awareness and acceptance of BFRBs, fostering a more inclusive and understanding environment for all affected.

Step 4: Replacement - Finding Alternative Behaviors

Replacing Body-Focused Repetitive Behaviors (BFRBs) with healthier alternatives is a crucial step in managing and reducing these behaviors. The goal is to redirect the urge to engage in BFRBs towards activities that provide similar sensory or emotional satisfaction without causing harm. By doing so, individuals can fulfill their needs in a more constructive manner, reducing the occurrence of BFRBs over time.

1. **Identifying Healthier Alternatives**

The first step in replacement is to identify activities that can effectively substitute Body-Focused Repetitive Behaviors (BFRBs). Start by considering what specific sensation or relief the BFRB provides. Is it a way to manage stress, cope with boredom, or fulfill a need for sensory stimulation? Once you've determined the underlying need, look for non-harmful activities that can replicate a similar feeling or satisfaction.

For instance, if skin picking is primarily driven by a need to keep your hands busy and provide tactile feedback, alternatives like squeezing a stress ball, using a fidget spinner, or engaging in craft activities like knitting or drawing can be beneficial.

These alternatives should not only replicate the sensory experience but also be easy to access, ensuring they are a practical choice when the urge arises. Additionally, they should be appealing enough to draw your attention away from the BFRB, ideally becoming a source of enjoyment and relaxation in their own right.

2. Implementing New Behaviors

Once suitable alternatives are identified, the next step is to implement them consistently. This involves integrating these activities into your daily routine, especially during times when you are most vulnerable to body-focused repetitive behaviors (BFRBs). Placing stress balls or fidget toys in accessible locations, such as your workspace, living area, or even your car, ensures they are readily available when the urge arises.

You might also consider carrying a small fidget toy in your pocket or bag for on-the-go use. Practice using these substitutes during moments of idle time, like waiting in line or during a commute, or in times of stress, such as before a big meeting or presentation, to build a habitual and effective response. Over time, these new habits can help reduce the frequency and intensity of BFRB urges, leading to a healthier and more mindful lifestyle.

3. Importance of Alternatives

Implementing alternative behaviors is essential because it provides a constructive outlet for the energy or emotion that drives BFRBs. By channeling these impulses into non-destructive activities, individuals can reduce the physical and emotional toll that BFRBs often entail. Alternatives help in breaking the automatic response cycle, allowing for more mindful engagement with one's actions.

4. **Examples of Effective Substitutes**

- **Tactile Alternatives**: Use items like stress balls, fidget cubes, or textured fabrics to occupy your hands. These tools can provide a satisfying sensory experience that helps distract from body-focused repetitive behaviors (BFRBs) by keeping your hands engaged.

- **Creative Activities**: Engage in activities such as drawing, knitting, or coloring. These hobbies not only keep your hands busy but also allow you to tap into your creativity and find relaxation through artistic expression. The focus required for these activities can divert your attention away from BFRBs and provide a sense of accomplishment.

- **Physical Movement**: Incorporate activities like yoga or stretching into your routine. These exercises engage both the body and the mind, offering a calming effect that can help manage stress and reduce the urge for BFRBs. Regular physical movement can also improve overall well-being and increase mindfulness.

- **Mindfulness Exercises**: Practice deep breathing or meditation techniques to center your thoughts and calm your mind. By focusing on your breath and being present in the moment, you can reduce stress and the compulsion to engage in BFRBs. Mindfulness exercises can serve as a powerful tool for managing anxiety and promoting mental clarity.

Finding and implementing alternative behaviors is a proactive approach to managing BFRBs. By understanding what needs the BFRBs fulfill, you can select purposeful substitutes that align with your lifestyle and preferences. This strategy not only reduces the frequency of BFRBs but also enhances overall well-being by promoting healthier habits and self-awareness. Through consistent practice, these alternatives can become a natural part of your coping toolkit, leading to lasting change.

Step 5: Support - Seeking Help from Professionals and Support Groups

Professional help can be instrumental in managing Body-Focused Repetitive Behaviors (BFRBs). Therapists and counselors provide valuable guidance tailored to your specific needs, helping you navigate the complexities of BFRBs with expert insight.

Engaging with a professional can offer a structured approach to understanding and addressing the psychological aspects of BFRBs, empowering you to adopt effective strategies for change.

1. **Cognitive-Behavioral Therapy (CBT)**

Cognitive-Behavioral Therapy (CBT) is a widely recognized and effective treatment for BFRBs. This therapy focuses on identifying and changing negative thought patterns and behaviors associated with BFRBs.

CBT helps individuals recognize triggers and develop coping mechanisms to reduce the urge to engage in repetitive behaviors. By working with a trained therapist, you can gain a deeper understanding of the cognitive processes that drive your actions and learn practical skills to manage them.

2. **Habit Reversal Training**

Habit Reversal Training (HRT) is another effective therapeutic approach for BFRBs. HRT involves increasing awareness of the behavior and its triggers, developing competing responses that are incompatible with the BFRB, and building motivation and support for behavior change. This structured method empowers individuals to substitute harmful habits with healthier alternatives, leading to a reduction in BFRBs over time.

3. The Role of Support Groups

Joining support groups can be incredibly beneficial for those dealing with BFRBs. These groups provide a safe space to share experiences and connect with others who understand the challenges you face.

By participating in support groups, you can gain insights from others' experiences, receive encouragement, and build a sense of community that reduces feelings of isolation. Sharing your journey with others can provide the motivation needed to continue striving for change.

5. Reducing Feelings of Isolation

Feeling connected to a community of individuals who share similar challenges can significantly reduce feelings of isolation. Support groups and peer networks offer an opportunity to exchange coping strategies, celebrate successes, and offer mutual support, fostering a sense of belonging and understanding. This connection can be a powerful motivator, reinforcing the belief that you are not alone and that change is possible.

Seeking support from professionals and joining support groups are crucial steps in managing BFRBs. Professional guidance through therapies like CBT and HRT provides effective tools for behavior change, while support groups offer community and encouragement.

Together, these resources can enhance your journey toward healing, helping you feel supported and motivated to achieve your goals. Embracing support not only facilitates personal growth but also contributes to a broader understanding and acceptance of BFRBs within the community.

Step 6: Practice - Implementing New Habits Consistently

Consistency is the cornerstone of forming new, healthier habits, especially when it comes to managing Body-Focused Repetitive Behaviors (BFRBs). Regular practice not only reinforces these new habits but also helps to gradually replace the old behaviors with positive alternatives. Establishing a consistent routine can create a sense of stability and progress, which is essential in sustaining change.

1. **Setting Realistic Goals**

To implement new habits effectively, it's crucial to set realistic and attainable goals. Start by defining small, manageable objectives that can be easily incorporated into your daily routine without overwhelming yourself.

For instance, if your aim is to replace skin picking with a less harmful activity, begin by committing to dedicating just a few minutes each day to this new behavior. Gradually increase the time as you become more accustomed and comfortable with the new habit, allowing it to naturally integrate into your lifestyle.

Additionally, break down your larger goals into smaller, actionable steps. This approach not only helps track progress but also maintains motivation by offering regular feelings of achievement. Remember that clear, achievable goals provide the necessary direction and make the overall process feel less daunting.

Celebrate small victories along the way to reinforce positive behavior and keep the momentum going. By focusing on manageable milestones, you set yourself up for long-term success in adopting healthier habits.

2. Celebrating Small Victories

Recognizing and celebrating small victories is vital in maintaining motivation throughout your personal or professional journey. Whether you are working towards a fitness goal, advancing in your career, or developing a new skill, each small achievement, no matter how minor it may seem, signifies progress and should be acknowledged. For example, if you're aiming to run a marathon, completing those first few miles without stopping is a small victory worth celebrating.

Celebrating these milestones fosters a positive mindset, boosts confidence, and reinforces your commitment to adopting healthier behaviors or habits. Acknowledging such achievements can take many forms, such as treating yourself to a nice meal, sharing your success with friends or family, or simply reflecting on your progress.

This acknowledgment can serve as a powerful motivator to continue striving towards your larger goals. By taking the time to appreciate these small wins, you build resilience and keep yourself focused on the broader vision you aim to achieve.

3. **The Role of Patience and Persistence**

Patience and persistence are key components of success when implementing new habits. Change is a gradual process, and it's important to acknowledge that setbacks may occur. These setbacks do not equate to failure; rather, they are opportunities for learning and growth. By maintaining a patient and persistent attitude, you allow yourself the grace to continue moving forward despite challenges, ultimately leading to long-term success in managing BFRBs.

By focusing on consistency, setting realistic goals, celebrating progress, and maintaining patience and persistence, you can effectively integrate new habits into your routine. These strategies will not only aid in managing BFRBs but also contribute to overall personal growth and resilience.

Step 7: Reflection - Monitoring Progress and Making Adjustments

Regular reflection is a powerful tool in for managing Body-Focused Repetitive Behaviors (BFRBs). It helps maintain awareness of your journey and keeps motivation high by allowing you to see the progress you've made.

By reflecting on both achievements and setbacks, you gain valuable insights into your behaviors and the effectiveness of the strategies you are using. This self-awareness is crucial for understanding which approaches are beneficial and which may need tweaking or replacing.

1. **Using a Journal for Tracking Progress**

A journal is an invaluable asset for tracking your progress with Body-Focused Repetitive Behaviors (BFRBs). It serves as a tangible record of your journey, documenting improvements, challenges, triggers, and emotional responses. By regularly recording your thoughts and experiences, you create a reflective space that can offer clarity and insight into your behaviors.

When using a journal, be consistent in your entries to capture a clear and comprehensive picture of your experiences over time. This practice not only helps identify patterns and triggers but also highlights the positive strides you have made.

Recognizing these achievements reinforces the importance of your efforts and dedication, reminding you of how far you've come and motivating you to continue on your path toward better management of BFRBs. Additionally, reviewing past entries can provide encouragement and a sense of accomplishment, as you witness your own growth and resilience in facing challenges.

2. **Adapting Strategies to Evolving Needs**

As you progress in your recovery journey, your needs and circumstances may evolve, necessitating thoughtful adjustments to your strategies. This evolution can be influenced by various factors, such as changes in your daily routine, mental well-being, or external stressors. Reflection becomes a crucial tool in this process, allowing you to assess which methods are proving effective and which might require modification or enhancement.

By taking the time to reflect, you can gain valuable insights into what works best for you personally and identify areas that need improvement or a different approach. Being flexible and open to change is vital in addressing your evolving needs, as it encourages a mindset that embraces growth and learning.

This adaptability ensures that your approach remains relevant and effective as you continue to work towards reducing Body-Focused Repetitive Behaviors (BFRBs), ultimately supporting your long-term goals and overall well-being.

By committing to regular reflection, utilizing a journal, and being willing to adapt your strategies, you can create a dynamic and responsive plan for managing BFRBs. These practices not only promote personal growth and self-awareness but also empower you to take charge of your recovery journey with confidence and resilience.

Applying the 7 Steps to Other BFRBs

1. **Flexibility in Approach**

Adapting the 7-step method designed initially for skin picking to other Body-Focused Repetitive Behaviors (BFRBs) like nail biting and hair pulling requires a flexible mindset. Each BFRB presents unique triggers and challenges, necessitating personalized approaches.

This adaptability is crucial in identifying and applying strategies that effectively address specific behaviors.

For instance, while skin picking may be addressed with certain tactile replacements or barriers, nail-biting might benefit from keeping nails trimmed or using bitter-tasting polish as a deterrent. Similarly, hair pulling might be mitigated through tactile interventions like wearing textured gloves. Understanding the distinct characteristics and triggers of each behavior ensures that the approach remains relevant and effective.

2. **Gradual Recovery Process**

Recognizing that recovery is a gradual and ongoing process is essential when applying these steps to various BFRBs. Patience and perseverance are your allies as you navigate the challenges of managing these behaviors. It's important to set realistic expectations and understand that progress may be slow but steady.

Embracing a patient mindset allows for reflection on progress and the making of necessary adjustments along the way. Perseverance is critical in overcoming setbacks, which are natural parts of the recovery journey.

By adapting strategies to suit the specific needs of different BFRBs, and maintaining a patient and persistent attitude, you enhance the likelihood of successfully managing and reducing these behaviors.

This approach not only facilitates recovery but also promotes personal growth and resilience, empowering you to take control of your journey with confidence.

Chapter 6: Creating a Sustainable Routine for Lasting Change

Creating lasting change requires a sustainable routine that supports the individual's goals and recovery. This chapter will explore practical strategies to maintain progress and prevent relapse.

Tips for Maintaining Progress and Preventing Relapse

To sustain change in managing Body-Focused Repetitive Behaviors (BFRBs), it's crucial to focus on consistency and vigilance. Here are some tips:

- **Set Achievable Goals**: Regularly set and review goals to keep your motivation high. Choose realistic objectives to foster a sense of accomplishment.

- **Identify Triggers**: Recognize potential triggers and prepare strategies to manage them, such as setting reminders or practicing mindfulness.

- **Learn from Setbacks**: Treat setbacks as learning opportunities rather than failures. Reflect on what happened and adapt your approach to strengthen your recovery.

Building a Supportive Environment and Lifestyle Changes

Creating a nurturing environment is vital for a successful recovery journey:

- **Cultivate Supportive Relationships**: Surround yourself with understanding and supportive individuals. Educate your friends and family about BFRBs to gain informed support.

- **Implement Lifestyle Changes**: Engage in regular exercise, maintain a balanced diet, and ensure you get enough sleep. These habits promote overall health, reducing the risk of relapse.

- **Modify Your Environment**: Declutter your space and remove items that might trigger BFRBs. A calming environment can enhance your recovery efforts.

Emphasizing Self-care and Self-Compassion in the Recovery Journey

Self-care and self-compassion are essential components of a sustainable routine:

- **Prioritize Self-Care**: Engage in activities that nourish your body and mind, such as yoga, meditation, or creative pursuits, to alleviate stress and build resilience.

- **Cultivate Self-Compassion**: Approach your journey with kindness and understanding. Acknowledge that recovery includes challenges, and avoid harsh self-criticism.

By integrating these strategies, you can develop a sustainable routine that not only supports long-term change and resilience in managing BFRBs but also enhances your overall well-being and personal growth.

Conclusion

Congratulations on reaching the end of this comprehensive guide on managing Body-Focused Repetitive Behaviors (BFRBs)! Your dedication to understanding and addressing these behaviors is a commendable step toward positive change and personal growth. As you reflect on the insights shared, let's explore how you can continue applying these strategies in your daily life, while maintaining a focus on empowerment and resilience.

Understanding BFRBs is about more than curbing behaviors; it's about embracing a holistic approach that nurtures both your mind and body. By recognizing these behaviors as more than just habits, you empower yourself to address the psychological and emotional triggers that underlie them. You've taken the time to educate yourself, which transforms how you view BFRBs—not as personal shortcomings, but as challenges that can be managed with the right tools and mindset.

Throughout this guide, you've explored strategies designed to help you take control. From understanding triggers and employing mindfulness techniques to seeking professional support and joining community groups, each step is crafted to help you build a personalized path to recovery. Implementing these strategies requires patience and persistence, yet the rewards are profound. By consistently practicing new habits, you establish a foundation for long-term well-being and resilience.

As you continue to apply these strategies, remember that change is a gradual process. Setbacks may occur, but they are not failures. They are opportunities to learn and adapt. Embrace each small victory, as these are the building blocks of sustainable change. Celebrate your progress, and don't hesitate to revisit your goals and strategies, refining them as necessary to suit your evolving needs.

Your path is uniquely yours, but you are never alone. Engaging with supportive communities and professionals can provide the encouragement and understanding you need. Sharing experiences with others who understand the challenges of BFRBs can be incredibly uplifting. It reminds you that you are part of a community of individuals dedicated to personal growth and resilience.

Self-care and self-compassion are crucial in this process. Prioritizing activities that nourish your soul and alleviate stress can build your resilience and enhance your quality of life. Whether through mindful practices like yoga and meditation or creative outlets that channel your energy positively, these activities help center you. They serve as a reminder that taking care of yourself is not just a part of recovery; it's a fundamental aspect of living a balanced life.

As you move forward, keep in mind the power of self-compassion. It's easy to fall into the trap of self-criticism, especially when faced with setbacks. However, treating yourself with kindness and understanding is essential. Recognize that everyone's path is different, and perfection is not the goal—progress is. Allow yourself the grace to make mistakes and learn from them, reinforcing your commitment to change.

The strategies outlined in this guide are tools for empowerment. They offer you the capability to transform your relationship with BFRBs, shifting from a state of struggle to one of understanding and control. By implementing these strategies, you are actively choosing to prioritize your mental and physical health, paving the way for a more fulfilling and confident version of yourself.

In essence, managing BFRBs is about reclaiming your sense of agency and embracing the possibility of change. It's about recognizing your strength and resilience and trusting in your ability to navigate challenges. By taking this step, you are investing in your future, one where BFRBs do not define you but are simply a part of your story.

Thank you for dedicating your time and energy to this guide. Your willingness to learn and grow is a testament to your strength. As you move forward, hold onto the insights and tools you've gathered here. Use them to build the life you envision—one filled with self-awareness, empowerment, and peace.

Remember, you have the power to create positive change. Embrace each day as an opportunity to apply what you've learned, and let your path be guided by hope, resilience, and the unwavering belief in your ability to thrive. You are capable, you are resilient, and you are not alone. Here's to your continued growth and success on this empowering path!

FAQ

What are Body-Focused Repetitive Behaviors (BFRBs) and how do they affect individuals?

BFRBs are compulsive actions like skin picking, nail-biting, and hair pulling that individual engage in often subconsciously. These behaviors can lead to physical harm, such as sores or hair loss, and emotional distress, including feelings of shame and anxiety. They can also affect daily life, impacting productivity, social interactions, and overall well-being.

What are the common triggers for BFRBs, and how can I identify mine?

Triggers can be emotional (stress, anxiety), situational (specific environments or activities), or sensory (physical sensations like rough skin). Identifying your triggers involves paying attention to when and where the behaviors occur and the emotions or situations associated with them. Keeping a journal can help track patterns and pinpoint specific triggers.

What strategies can help in managing and reducing BFRBs?

Effective strategies include behavioral interventions like Habit Reversal Training (HRT), mindfulness practices, and cognitive-behavioral therapy (CBT). Replacing the repetitive behavior with healthier alternatives, such as using fidget toys, and seeking support from professionals and support groups can also be beneficial.

How can mindfulness help in managing BFRBs?

Mindfulness increases awareness of your thoughts and actions, helping you recognize triggers and urges before they lead to BFRBs. By practicing techniques such as meditation and deep breathing, you can learn to pause and choose healthier responses, reducing the frequency and severity of your behaviors.

What role does self-care play in managing BFRBs?

Self-care is crucial as it helps reduce stress and build resilience, which can decrease the urge to engage in BFRBs. Activities like regular exercise, adequate rest, and engaging in hobbies or relaxation techniques can support mental and physical health, aiding recovery.

Are there any tools or apps that can assist in managing BFRBs?

Yes, habit-tracking apps can be useful for logging behaviors, identifying patterns, and setting goals. Many apps also offer reminders, motivational messages, and online communities for support, helping maintain accountability and motivation.

What should I do if I experience setbacks in managing my BFRBs?

Setbacks are a natural part of the recovery process. It's important to view them as learning opportunities rather than failures. Reflect on what triggered the setback, adjust your strategies as needed, and continue to practice self-compassion and patience. Seeking support from professionals or support groups can also provide encouragement and guidance.

References and Helpful Links

Dermatillomania (Skin picking). (2024, May 1). Cleveland Clinic. https://my.clevelandclinic.org/health/diseases/22706-dermatillomania-skin-picking

International OCD Foundation. (2022, November 29). *International OCD Foundation | What is Skin Picking Disorder?* https://iocdf.org/about-ocd/related-disorders/skin-picking-disorder/

The TLC Foundation for Body-Focused Repetitive Behaviors. (n.d.). *Body-Focused Repetitive Behavior | BFRB | BFRB Awareness*. https://www.bfrb.org/your-journey/what-is-a-bfrb

How to treat skin picking disorder (Excoriation). (2024, February 8). WebMD. https://www.webmd.com/mental-health/skin-picking-disorder

Phillips, K. A., & Stein, D. J. (2023, July 12). *Body-Focused Repetitive Behavior Disorder*. Merck Manual Consumer Version. https://www.merckmanuals.com/home/mental-health-disorders/obsessive-compulsive-and-related-disorders/body-focused-repetitive-behavior-disorder#:~:text=People%20with%20body%2Dfocused%20repetitive%20behavior%20disorder%20compulsively%20pick%2C%20pull,also%20body%2Dfocused%20repetitive%20behaviors.

A complete Guide to Body-Focused Repetitive Behavior | Brain Balance. (n.d.). https://www.brainbalancecenters.com/blog/body-focused-repetitive-behavior#:~:text=Body%2Dfocused%20repetitive%20behaviors%20are,lips%2C%20cheeks%2C%20or%20tongue.

Okumuş, H. G., & Akdemir, D. (2022). Body Focused Repetitive Behavior Disorders: behavioral models and neurobiological mechanisms. *Turkish Journal of Psychiatry*. https://doi.org/10.5080/u26213

www.ingramcontent.com/pod-product-compliance
Lightning Source LLC
LaVergne TN
LVHW012046070526
838201LV00079B/3706